TIMOTHY BEATY

Childhood Asthma

A Practical Guide For Parents

This book is dedicated to my supportive and lovely wife, my four charming children, and the patients who have taught me about strength and courage just as much as I have taught them about their health.

Contents

1

Introduction

As a pediatric pulmonologist, I have had the great privilege of helping thousands of children and their families understand and manage their asthma. The story is usually the same. There is fear, anxiety, and confusion regarding asthma. Most parents hold back their questions at first, but as trust grows, the questions begin to come. Does my child have asthma? Will they outgrow it? How do I use these inhalers? Why do I need the inhaler when the nebulizer works so much better? Asthma is like a boa constrictor waiting behind every minor cold, sporting event, and family gathering, ready to take your breath away.

I schedule new patient consultations for 90 minutes. Ninety minutes is a luxury that most pediatricians cannot offer their patients. In truth, even 90 minutes is not always enough time. Even with as many patients as I have treated, understanding any individual family's struggles always requires investments of time, interest, and empathy. I have seen so many families' anxieties melt away as I explained the same topics covered in this book, powerful proof that there is a great need for a practical guide of asthma for parents who just want their kids to be well. Parents want to understand what is happening to their child, and how to help them be well.

This book will not be filled with statistics and clinical trial results. I must admit, there may be statements in this book that are not 100% true *(ok, there are some statistics).* The intention of this book is to give you a practical understanding of asthma and how to manage it. There are times when I sacrifice accuracy for usefulness and practicality.

The stories and examples in this book are pulled from my experience and interactions with hundreds of families like yours through the last ten years. I have had to test my teaching and approach against the realities of caring for a child with asthma. Over time, only the most useful strategies remain. The lessons contained in this book are those that I believe have the greatest impact on my patients' lives. I pray it will have a similar impact on yours.

2

Asthma Effects Children - And Their Families

There it is. That cough. It always starts with the cough. Most parents wouldn't even notice, but you do. That cough predicts another restless night, maybe a trip to the emergency room. It was just an innocent trip to the park - why does it always go like this?

Of course, the doctors gave you these inhalers. They're supposed to help. Do you use the blue one or the orange one first? Will he even be able to breathe well enough to take it? You know exactly what will happen. He will be ok as you put him to bed. Then at 12:30 AM you hear the cough and gasping. You'll see his ribs and stomach moving as he struggles for air. Nothing works, so you go to the emergency room where it is always the same - the nebulizer, tubes, wires, and another restless night. They'll see his oxygen is low and slap a cannula on his nose. The nebulizer does work, but it may take 2-3 treatments. A steroid shot and prescription, and it's back home - if you're lucky.

Why does it always have to be like this? That cough... that asthma.

Asthma Background

Asthma is the most common chronic disease among children in developed nations. I promised this book would not be about statistics, but some numbers are too impressive to omit. In the United States, about 5 million children, or 1 in 12, have asthma. These children account for more than 700,000 emergency room visits, 74,000 hospitalizations, and - unfortunately - 100 deaths annually. Even without severe attacks, asthma accounts for over 10 million missed school days per year, not to mention missed work days and increased cost of childcare for their parents.

On the other hand, asthma is an imminently treatable condition. I have had the privilege of helping thousands of parents just like you replace their confusion and anxiety with knowledge and confidence. I will not waste your time with jargon, statistics, and scientific graphs. Instead, I have distilled these concepts down to their most important points, which you can use today, and every day, to help your child thrive despite their asthma.

3

What is Asthma?

Asthma is a clinical diagnosis. That means that there is no test to diagnose asthma. Asthma is a story that takes place over time. If the story contains two primary elements, it is likely a story about asthma. Those elements are:

1. Recurrent or chronic coughing and wheezing
2. Symptoms improve with bronchodilators (ie, albuterol - see Chapter 3)

Albuterol is a very specific medicine. There are dozens of reasons to cough, and albuterol only treats one of those - an asthma cough. When someone asks me if they have asthma, my #1 question is, "Does albuterol help?" If so, there is a high likelihood that we are dealing with asthma. It is important to note that by "help," I mean that albuterol relieves your symptoms in a way that makes sense for how it works. The benefit will be evident in around 10 minutes and last for around 60-90 minutes, even if the symptoms return after that.

There are supporting elements that make the story more convincing.

These are:

1. Symptoms are "triggered" by common stimuli (e.g., weather, exposures, exercise...)
2. Symptoms occur even outside of any known respiratory illness (i.e., a cold)
3. The child has known or suspected environmental allergies, such as dust mites.
4. The child has had eczema (atopic dermatitis)
5. The child's family has a history of asthma or allergies.

Certainly, a child with asthma can have none of these secondary elements, but it is uncommon.

As you can see, allergies play a major role in much of childhood asthma. Allergies also play a role in adult asthma, though to a lesser degree. Next, we'll talk about the link between allergies and asthma.

Why Do We Wheeze?

Just like our noses, our airways can react to allergens in the air. When we breathe, the air passes through our nose, sinus, windpipe (trachea), and into the lung. The windpipe splits into airways that take the air to the right and left lungs. After that, the airway split 26 more times to carry the air into all the different parts of the lung, with the tunnels getting smaller at each split. The inner lining of those airways is similar to the inner lining of the nose - that moist pink stuff that makes mucus sometimes. So, just like your nose, your airways will sometimes get swollen and congested, increasing their mucous production.

There is a difference between the airways in your lungs and your nose.

Your airways have an extra layer that is a muscle called the bronchial smooth muscles. These muscles surround the airways, and they have an important job. Their job is to *protect* your lung! They do this through a process called bronchoconstriction.

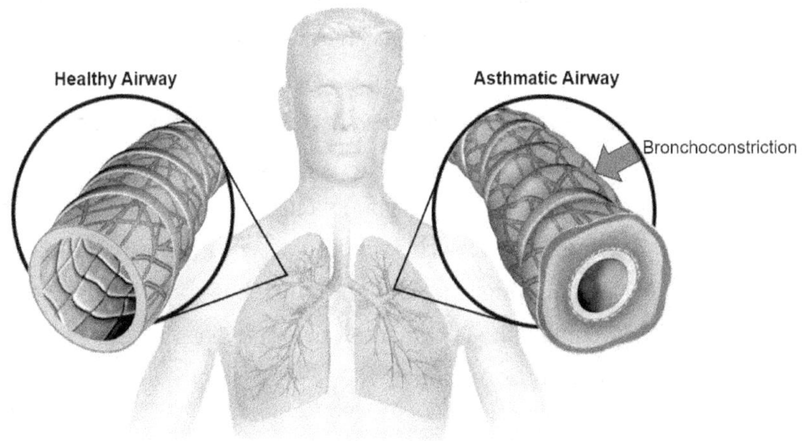

Healthy Airways compared to Asthmatic Airways

When your lung senses something dangerous in the air, such as burning ash, the airway muscles contract and squeeze the airways, making the tunnels smaller and tighter, just like a boa constrictor. This is called bronchoconstriction. Bronchoconstriction makes it hard to breathe. You may feel tightness or burning in the chest. Some children have described it to me as a rubber band around or an elephant sitting on your chest. One child told me it felt like a hamster sitting on his chest! Bronchoconstriction is also what causes wheezing - the whistling sound that air makes as it passes through those tight tunnels.

Bronchoconstriction also causes a cough reflex. Your body wants to cough because it wants whatever caused the bronchoconstriction, the dangerous stuff in the air, out of your body!

This would be normal in a burning building. People would be clutching their chests, coughing, and wheezing. They're not having an asthma attack - those airway muscles are doing the right thing! They are trying to protect the lung from the burning ash and hot air.

Now, imagine a 12-year-old who has cat allergies, but otherwise is completely well. He then visits his grandmother's house and finds 7 cats in the living room. Likely, you will next see him clutching his chest, coughing, and wheezing - exactly like if he was in a burning building! The cat hair he was inhaling was not dangerous, but his body reacted to it just like the burning ash. The normal, protective reflex has become over-active because of his cat allergy.

I can just sense many of you nodding your heads in understanding now. However, some of you are thinking, "But doc, my kid doesn't have any allergies. We've even been tested for allergies THREE TIMES!"

Non-Allergic Asthma

You are 100% correct. There are children with asthma who do not have allergies. However, because they have asthma, by definition, they will experience the same symptoms - recurrent coughing and wheezing that improves with albuterol.

Bronchoconstriction can occur with any trigger or exposure that the lung might sense as dangerous. Common triggers of non-allergic asthma include viral infections (ie, colds), exercise, cigarette smoke, even temperature changes! I love to ask teenagers if they cough when eating cold foods since so many suddenly realize that they do! I suspect this is because the simple act of swallowing frozen foods like ice cream changes the temperature inside the chest, stimulating asthma symptoms.

In short, any change or irritant in the air you are breathing could cause bronchoconstriction. This may all seem scary, but now we are getting to the good part.

4

Asthma Trigger Worksheet

List your child's triggers here.

It may be helpful to consider what happened during or prior to your child's major asthma attacks. These may include seasons, holidays, trips, field trips, exposure to animals, exposure to blooming trees or cut grass, weather changes, activities, etc.

____

____

____

____

____

5

Asthma Treatment

Once doctors make an asthma diagnosis, they will next attempt to categorize it by severity. The details of this are outside the scope of this guidebook, but some explanation will be helpful for you. Your doctor will assess two things:

1. Risk: How often you have attacks that require care in an emergency room, hospital, or intensive care unit.
2. Impairment: How is your asthma affecting your daily life. For example, are you limited in sports*, do you depend on albuterol to complete daily tasks, etc.

* Side note: I just triggered Some of you by saying "limited in sports." Have no fear. None (zero, zilch) of my patients should be limited in their sports participation. I tell my patients, "if you are limited in sports because of your asthma, it does NOT mean that you quit the sport. It means that I need to do my job better. It may take me a while to get you there, but I will get

you there."

Once your asthma severity has been assessed, there are guidelines to help guide initial treatments. You will likely be prescribed a "controller therapy" to help reduce your risk and impairment. The guidelines will recommend reassessing your risk and impairment after you have been on the controller therapy for 1–3 months. This is because the controller therapies are usually starting to show their effectiveness after two weeks of consistent use.

Yes – I said *weeks*. Asthma is a great lesson in patience and faith for parents. Your child's asthma has likely been brewing for months and years, it will take weeks or months for us to get it under control. But be encouraged – we will.

What is "Well-Controlled" Asthma?

Once your child is on a controller therapy, it does not necessarily mean they need that controller indefinitely. The goal of treatment is to keep your child "well-controlled." The actual definition of well-controlled may differ for individual situations, but in general well-controlled means:

1. Using albuterol <2 days per week
2. Waking from sleep with asthma symptoms <2 times per month
3. Participating in physical activity without restrictions*
4. Avoiding emergency room visits, hospitalizations, or extra medicines like steroids for asthma attacks.

*If taking albuterol prior to or before exercises resolves symptoms, it still counts as well-controlled.

If your child is still not well-controlled, increasing your controller dose or switching to another controller will be recommended. Per national and international guidelines, decreasing your controller therapy is considered after at least three months of well-controlled asthma. That may include STOPPING your controller therapy in certain situations. We do this carefully. For instance, it may be unwise to stop a child's controller therapy in July when they are going to start school in August. You can bet with near certainty they will be home with an illness the second week of August!

How to Talk to Your Doctor

Today, doctors are more hurried than ever. While the complexity of medical care and treatment options has been expanding, the time physicians can spend with patients is actually dropping. Your doctor most likely wants to spend more time with you, but cannot due to time constraints and other obligations. A recent report found that primary care doctors need more than 24 hours in a day to provide all of the recommended care for their patients. Unless we all move to Jupiter or Elon Musk discovers a way to slow down the rotation of the Earth, that isn't happening.

Physicians are also bombarded with information daily. Physicians are trained to be able to take in large amounts of information, filter out what is useful, and discard the rest. You probably talk to your doctor the way you talk to everyone, with narratives. You tell them stories about your child's asthma attack on the playground or on a family trip. You want to tell him how scary it was. You want to tell him the doctors weren't sure if it was asthma or a cold, and everything seemed confused. Your doctor cares about these things, but the small details that make for a good story are often useless for developing a treatment plan. Your doctor is looking for specific pieces of information:

1. Current treatment plan
2. Adherence to the treatment plan (ie, are you frequently missing doses or taking your medicine improperly?)
3. The frequency and severity of asthma attacks
4. How your asthma affects your quality of life – your pain points you most want help with

The doctor wants to know what you are doing now and if it is working. If not, why isn't it working? Is it the wrong medicine or the right medicine being used improperly?

In Chapter 14 I will list further tips for questions to bring up with your physician.

Medications for Asthma

What Exactly is Albuterol?

Albuterol is the primary treatment for *the symptoms* of asthma. Albuterol is not a steroid. It is in a class of medicines called "beta agonists." More specifically, it is a "short acting beta agonist," or SABA. Albuterol is available in multiple forms, whether oral as a syrup, nebulized as a liquid, or in an inhaler. Oral albuterol is not recommended for use in the United States due to being less effective for asthma while also giving increased side effects. Side effects of albuterol include jitters, fast heart rates, and light-headedness.

You may have a closely related medication called levalbuterol. To make things more confusing, outside of the USA, albuterol is commonly known as "salbutamol." I will only use the word albuterol moving forward. You should take my use of albuterol as "nebulized or inhaled albuterol/levalbuterol/salbutamol." This book gives general information on how these medicines are used, but you should follow your physician's instructions for specifics.

Albuterol acts to relieve bronchoconstriction, thereby relieving the symptoms of asthma. Once the airways relax and open up, you will feel less chest tightness and shortness of breath. The cough reflex of bronchoconstriction will also resolve. Albuterol is not a "cough medicine." It will not help other kinds of cough. For instance, if your throat is sore and causing you to cough, albuterol will not help. On the other hand, albuterol WILL help your cough if you are having bronchoconstriction. We sometimes call albuterol a "rescue" medicine, since you use it to rescue you from asthma symptoms.

The problem with albuterol, as you have probably noticed, is twofold:

1. It is short-acting (60-240 minutes)
2. It does not treat the underlying cause of the bronchospasm - inflammation

This means that albuterol is very good at treating the symptoms of asthma, but it is not very good at preventing symptoms. If the albuterol is only going to last for 1-2 hours, you cannot give the albuterol at 8 AM and send your child off to school. By 10 AM it will be out of their system and no longer protecting them.

The answer is NOT to schedule albuterol every few hours. Albuterol is one of those medications that can stop working if used repetitively, a process called tachyphylaxis. When someone has tachyphylaxis to albuterol, their symptoms are very difficult to control. I do not want you to be scared to use your albuterol - if you need albuterol for symptoms, use it! But I do not want you over-using or becoming dependent on albuterol to get through your daily life. That puts you at risk for tachyphylaxis.

Most families who enter my clinic feel that nebulized albuterol works better than albuterol from an inhaler. There are multiple reasons for this, including that most emergency rooms still give nebulized albuterol, even for mild symptoms. However, albuterol is the same whether given by nebulization or inhaler.

I tell my patients that using an inhaler will not *feel* as good as giving the nebulizer. Some of this is mental. It simply feels better and more impressive to pull out "the machine" that makes noise and smoke, especially when your child is struggling to breathe. You get to see it work. This is a placebo effect. Your child may also be benefiting from having to sit and breathe quietly for 10-15 minutes, but you can have them do this without a nebulizer. There are some real differences between nebulized and albuterol from an inhaler that will be helpful for you to know.

First, albuterol takes about 5-15 minutes to start working. Because a nebulized albuterol treatment also takes about 10 minutes, by the end of the treatment you are already seeing the albuterol effects. An inhaler will take a minute or less for the whole treatment, but your child will still be struggling and coughing his/her head off for another 5-10 minutes. When this happens, your brain will naturally panic and start telling you that the inhaler is not working - "Go get the machine!" In other words, using an inhaler is so much faster that you need to be MORE patient -

you won't see if it helped for about 10 minutes.

Systemic Steroids:

Asthma attacks are generally treated by systemic steroids given by mouth, injection, or intravenously. I will use the term 'systemic steroids' for this treatment to differentiate these medications from other kinds of steroids. The primary systemic steroids used for asthma are prednisone/prednisolone and dexamethasone. Systemic steroids treat asthma attacks by reducing airway inflammation and edema, thereby reducing the tendency to bronchoconstriction.

Systemic steroids work well to treat asthma, at the risk of side effects. As you have probably noticed, short courses of systemic steroids turn your kids into angry, hungry, bouncing balls of energy, but do not generally cause any lasting adverse effects. On the other hand, chronic or frequent use of steroids will almost certainly cause side effects. Systemic steroid side effects are bad news: obesity, diabetes, stunted growth, osteoporosis, acne, cataracts, etc., all kinds of things you do not want for your child! For children who will have multiple asthma attacks per year, relying on albuterol and systemic steroids is not a good plan. We need an alternative to keep your child out of the emergency room and off systemic steroids.

Asthma Controllers

To help reduce the frequency and severity of asthma attacks, doctors will frequently prescribe controller therapies. These medications reduce airway inflammation or prevent bronchospasm without the risk of systemic steroids or albuterol tachyphylaxis.

Inhaled Corticosteroids (ICS): These are steroid inhalers. The steroid in these medications reduces inflammation in the airways, reducing the risk of bronchoconstriction. Although these medications are steroids, most people have no real risk of steroid side effects with ICS. Partly, this is because the dose of steroids in these inhalers is minuscule compared to systemic steroids. Notice that ICS are dosed in mcg – that's MICROgrams. A microgram is 1/1000th of a milligram (mg).

Warning: There is a little bit of math here

Consider a 40 lb child with an asthma attack. His dose of prednisone is 40 mg daily. Forty milligrams convert to 40,000 micrograms! He swallows the 40,000 mcg and almost all of it is absorbed it into the bloodstream. Some prednisone goes to the lungs to reduce inflammation, but the rest circulates throughout the body. That circulation is where the side effects come from.

Most children with asthma who are 40 lb would do just fine with fluticasone 110mcg, 2 puffs twice daily, or 440 mcg. Compared to 40,000 mcg for prednisone - the dose of fluticasone is tiny! To make things even better, only 10-20% of the inhaled steroid is absorbed into the bloodstream.

ICS and height reduction: You will likely see warnings that inhaled steroids can affect your child's height. That is true. However, this was primarily seen in young girls who were on high-dose ICS for three years consecutively. They had height reduction that persisted into adulthood, but it was only 1.1 cm, less than half an inch. More often, studies show that children's growth does slow for the first few months after starting an ICS compared to children on a placebo. However, they soon catch up and return to their natural growth curve. Both of these effects on height are much less significant than having severe asthma attacks and requiring high doses of systemic steroids.

ICS have other potential side effects. There is a risk of thrush, sore throat, or even voice changes if the inhaled steroid stays in the mouth. These can be prevented by simply rinsing the medication out of the mouth after inhaling. I tell my patients to brush their teeth, and the dentist and I are happy! Further side effects are less common and should be discussed with your physician.

ICS are prescribed as once or twice/day inhalations. That means you use them whether you are well or sick. Currently, the only group of people who would use ICS on an "as needed" basis are young children aged 0-4 years of age. Since those patients often only have symptoms during respiratory infections, some can prevent or reduce their asthma exacerbations by only starting ICS at the onset of respiratory infection. The idea is that they don't need a daily anti-inflammatory medicine, but as soon as the respiratory infection starts, you need a very high anti-inflammatory to the airways to prevent the infection from going to the chest.

Long Acting Beta Agonists (LABA): These medications have a similar effect as albuterol to relax the airways, but last for a much longer period of time. In the USA, these medications are only available in combination with an ICS. When LABA were used without an inhaled steroid, it actually increased the risk of a serious asthma attack - you really need the anti-inflammatory effect of the ICS for the LABA to help you with your symptoms.

Recent asthma treatment guidelines have recommended some patients use what is called SMART, or Single Maintenance and Reliever Therapy. This means they have a combined ICS-LABA inhaler that they use as both their controller and rescue medicine. This is only possible with certain LABA, so you should not use this without your doctor's instructions. There are a few benefits to this strategy. First, there is only one inhaler to keep up with rather than separate inhalers for controllers and rescue. Second, as your child needs his rescue medicine, he is also increasing his treatment with the ICS, helping to reduce the inflammation as it is flaring.

The problem with SMART currently is that most ICS-LABA inhalers are designed to have just enough medication to use as a controller for one month. If you also use extra doses for rescue, you will run out of medication too quickly. I suspect payers and pharmaceutical companies will develop solutions for this in the future.

Leukotriene Receptor Antagonists (LTRA): These are medicines that block the action of chemicals in our body involved in inflammation called leukotrienes. The primary LTRA used in children at the time of this writing is called montelukast. It is one of America's most commonly used medications because it is easy to take and helps many conditions, including allergies, asthma, and snoring. It is even FDA-approved for exercise-induced asthma in children. Montelukast is usually used as a secondary or additional controller in for people who are not well-controlled with an inhaled corticosteroid alone.

The most concerning side effect of montelukast is behavior and mood disturbance. It can cause toddlers to have nightmares or worsening tantrums. In teenagers sometimes it can lead to depressed moods and has been linked to suicidal behavior. Discussing these issues with your physician is vitally important, especially if your child has mood or mental health concerns.

Miscellaneous Therapies: I have now covered the primary medications used in childhood asthma. Asthma therapies are constantly being developed, so it would be impossible to list them all in this guidebook. I will list a few here, but you will need to discuss them with your physician for details.

Allergy desensitization can be helpful in treating allergic asthma, particularly for people with only a few (or even one) allergen sensitivities. A developing class of medications called "biologic" therapies is emerging to treat people with severe, uncontrolled asthma. These medications are monoclonal antibodies or small molecules used to reduce the inflammatory pathways in the body. Because these therapies are expensive and given by recurring injections, they are used in children with severe asthma that otherwise could not be controlled. These medications may become a preferred treatment for asthma since their anti-inflammatory effect may be superior to that of ICS. Before this happens, they must become cheaper and, ideally, have non-injectable formulations.

6

Your Child's Medication Worksheet

List your child's medications here. You can use this page to track therapy changes over time or as a discussion starter with your physician.

____

____

____

____

7

Will my child outgrow their asthma?

I could be asked this question multiple times per day. Unfortunately, since I cannot tell the future, it is not a question I can answer with certainty and still be truthful. Some people experience asthma symptoms for a period of life, and then the symptoms resolve for another period. If the patient is still a baby or toddler without any sign of allergies, there is a fairly good chance they will totally outgrow their asthma. For older children, I do suspect that the inflammation remains throughout their life, but it becomes less and less potent to the point it no longer causes symptoms. Because I do not treat adults, I do not have any direct experience with symptoms that recur later in life. For women, there is a tendency to develop asthma symptoms during pregnancy.

Another key thing to know is that our asthma controller therapies do not currently change the directory of the disease. You are not more likely to "outgrow" asthma by taking your medicines religiously. Similarly, taking asthma controllers is not going to make you "dependent" on them. The utility of these medications is that they keep your symptoms under control so that you can live your life and face less risk of emergency room visits and systemic steroid bursts.

8

How do I use this thing, anyway?

Inhaled medications may seem tricky at first, but I have never cared for a patient we couldn't find an effective option. It is important to remember that all of these inhaled medications are actually "topical," meaning they work by landing on the inside of the airways, just like if you were rubbing a steroid cream on an itchy rash. The only difference is the medicine particles need to be able to get all the way down to the lung before they land.

Nebulizers

Most children will begin their asthma treatments with a nebulizer. A nebulizer is the simplest method since all your child will need to do is breathe. The downside of nebulizers is their size, bulk, lack of portability, and the need for a power source. Further, the more effective controller therapies are only available in inhaler form.

The nebulizer is simple to use. I will describe the basic process here, but you should refer to the instructions provided with your device.

1. Plug in the compressor (the machine part)
2. Connect the tubing and nebulizer cup
3. Pour the medication solution into the nebulizer cup (mixing in saline if necessary)
4. Connect the mouthpiece or mask to the nebulizer cup
5. Place the mask on your child's face or mouthpiece in their mouth
6. Turn on the machine
7. Have your child take slow breaths.
8. The treatment is done with all the medication in the cup is gone. There will be no more mist coming out. You may need to tap the nebulizer cup to get drops of medicine down to the bottom of the cup.

You should wash the nebulizer cup and mouthpiece/mask with dish soap and warm water after each use, or disinfect as per the manufacturer recommendations. The timing for replacing the nebulizer, tubing, mask/mouthpiece, and compressor varies based on how frequently the device is used. In general, if the pieces are beginning to look worn out, ask your doctor for a new nebulizer kit.

Inhalers

The world is more complex than it used to be. There are now multiple styles of inhalers. Some inhalers will look like classic inhalers with a canister that you press to expel medicine out of the inhaler. Others will have nothing to press and are "breath actuated," meaning they detect when your inhalation and release the medicine. Some inhalers have a spacer device already connected, while others do not even expel the medication. Instead, they contain the medicine in capsules and dry powder that you inhale.

Fortunately, it is now easier than ever to find instructions on how to use your inhaler. Instructions will certainly come with your inhaler, but a simple internet search for your specific inhaler type will result in multiple results with specific instructions. It is outside of the scope of this guidebook to contain specific methods for every type of inhaler device.

I do want to point out some important points. If your inhaler has a canister to push, you will need to shake the inhaler vigorously ~10 times. If the inhaler has not been used in 2 weeks, go ahead and "prime" the inhaler by compressing the canister twice. This ensures there is active medication in the nozzle ready to help you. Never use an expired inhaler.

Spacers - Yes, you should use them!

There is one more important topic I cannot stress enough - spacers. I recommend spacers for all children under 12 years of age, and they can be helpful at any age. The spacer takes decreases the need for perfect inhalation and coordination. Essentially, if your child can breathe, they can take an inhaled medicine using a spacer.

Spacers also increase the amount of medication that reaches the lung. If you have ever sprayed an inhaler into the air, you will see that the medication particles come out in a cloud. Some particles move fast, and some are slow. Some particles go straight up or down. If you think about spraying that cloud into your mouth, some of the medication immediately hits your cheeks, the roof of the mouth, or tongue and is wasted. Fast-moving medicine particles experience turbulence, spin in the air, and land before they reach your lungs.

Spacers solve these problems by suspending the medicine particles into the air inside the spacer and slowing down the particles so they go down *smoothly*. For you physicists, this is called laminar flow. There are two primary methods for using a spacer.

Use the single breath and hold for children who can hold their breath for 10 seconds:

1. Attach the inhaler to the back end of the spacer
2. Take a deep breath, then exhale fully
3. Place the mouthpiece or mask on your face
4. Puff the medication
5. Inhale slowly, filling your lungs as much as possible
6. A whistling sound means that you are breathing too quickly - the air will be turbulent, affecting how much medicine gets to your lung.
7. Once you have the maximum amount of air, hold your breath for 10 seconds.
8. Exhale, catch your breath, and prepare for the next puff if needed.
9. A whistling sound means that you are breathing too quickly - the air will be turbulent, affecting how much medicine gets to your lung.

By doing this, the medication particles are slowed and suspended inside the spacer. The deep breath moves the particles down into the lungs. Because you're breathing slowly, there is less turbulence, and more particles reach your lungs. Finally, while you're holding your breath, the medication is landing.

For children who cannot hold their breath for 10 seconds, try the tidal breathing technique:

1. Attach the inhaler to the back end of the spacer
2. Take a deep breath, then exhale fully
3. Place the mouthpiece or mask on your face
4. Puff the medication
5. Take 6-10 slow, deep breaths.
6. If your spacer has a valve, the breaths should be strong enough to move the valve 6-10 times.
7. A whistling sound means that you are breathing too quickly - the air will be turbulent, affecting how much medicine gets to your lung.

You can wash a spacer with dish soap and warm water. Remember to let it air-dry. Do not wipe the inside of the spacer. If you wipe the inside of the spacer dry it may create a static cling that causes the medicine to stick to the spacer rather than move to your lung.

What if I miss a dose?

You will get the most benefit from your controller therapies if you follow your asthma action plan without missing doses. However, life happens, and we all miss doses from time to time. If you have a daily medication and missed your dose, I recommend taking the dose whenever you remember. You can then start back on your regular schedule the next day. If you are on a twice/day medication and are only late 4-6 hours for a dose, it is ok to take the dose and continue with the next dose as scheduled. If you are more than 6 hours late on your dose, go ahead and skip it. You can get back on schedule with your next dose. Some situations may be special, so ask your physician if he agrees with that plan. Most people will not be on a controller therapy more often than twice per day.

9

Lung Function Testing

L ung function is an important part of asthma management. A common misperception is that lung function testing can diagnose asthma - it does not. People can have asthma and still have normal lung function, and people without asthma can have abnormal lung function. We primarily use lung function testing, specifically a test called spirometry, to track asthma control over time.

Spirometry is a simple test to perform, but it is not easy. Spirometry measures someone's Forced Vital Capacity (FVC). The person will fill their lungs with air as much as possible, then exhale as hard as possible for as long as possible - until their lungs are completely empty, followed by a rapid inhalation. The exhalation should be at least 6 seconds, although for young children a 3 second exhalation can be accepted if everything else looks accurate. Then the child will need to repeat the test several more times until we can be sure they are consistent (at least three efforts). As you can imagine, this test requires patience and self-control, so we do not routinely order it on children less than six years of age.

10

Lung Function Test Log

If your child has performed lung functions, you can track their FEV1 here. You should also record the controller therapy they were on at the time:

Date	FEV1/FVC (<0.8 suggests asthma)	FEV1 % predicted (>80% normal)	Controller

11

How to Handle an Asthma Attack

I f your child has asthma, you will eventually deal with an asthma attack. I tell my patients that I cannot prevent their child from getting sick. A child in school can have anywhere from 4-12 colds per year and still be normal! My job is to get their asthma so well-controlled that when they do get sick, it is miserable for 3-5 days, and they will need albuterol. However, they will have avoided the emergency room and recovered in less than 1-2 weeks without systemic steroids.

When your child begins to get sick, follow your asthma action plan. It will likely instruct you to continue your controller therapy and use albuterol for symptoms. When your child has coughing, wheezing, or shortness of breath, start your albuterol as directed by your asthma action plan and assess if it is helping. If albuterol does help, be ready to continue giving it every 4 hours or so for the next two days, then less often as the symptoms improve. As long as you can manage the symptoms at home with albuterol, you do not necessarily need to ask for a steroid burst. In fact, they goal is to get through most of your illnesses without steroids.

Your albuterol most likcly has been prescribed to be given "every four hours as needed." We prescribe albuterol every four hours because needing it more often is a strong predictor for serious or fatal asthma attacks. You can use albuterol more often than every four hours, but it should only be done under the direction of a healthcare provider.

Many patients have asked me when they should take their child to the emergency room. The real answer is "If you are worried, you should take them." This is especially true for infants and young children who decompensate faster than older children. However, some general principles for making a trip to the emergency room include:

1. Struggling to breathe that does not improve 10-20 minutes after albuterol
2. Severe "retractions," or sinking in of the areas above and below the chest and ribs.
3. Your child cannot talk in full sentences, even after albuterol has taken effect
4. Persistent coughing and wheezing that you cannot control
5. They appear fatigued from breathing so hard
6. You notice color change like blue or grey lips/fingertips

12

Your Child's Exacerbations Diary

Keep track of ER visits, Hospitalizations, and steroid bursts here. Ideally, you will see this occur less and less with time! At worst, you may be able to spot patterns to help prevent exacerbations in the future.

____

____

____

____

13

Special Situations

Babies and toddlers

While asthma primarily affects school-age children with allergies, babies and toddlers can exhibit asthma symptoms. The difference is the cause of wheezing. Rather than allergies, babies and toddlers primarily wheeze in response to their frequent viral infections. Around 40% of children in America will have wheezing with an illness at least once in their life. Most of them will not go on to have asthma.

Any viral infection can cause wheezing, but Respiratory Syncytial Virus (RSV) is the major culprit. Eight out of 10 children in America will have had RSV by the time they are 2 years of age. For most of them, RSV is just a bad cold, but it is the one most likely to go to the chest and cause wheezing. The younger the child, the more likely RSV will cause a wheezing illness. This is called "bronchiolitis," and is different than "bronchitis" which is a generic term for an infection of the airways.

Wheezing in babies without viral infections is often due to airway irritants like secondhand tobacco smoke or aspiration (food, stomach contents, or other materials spilling into the lungs). Aspiration can occur both while eating or refluxing. Babies born prematurely wheeze more often than children born at term for multiple reasons, especially in the first 1-2 years of life. If a child is going to outgrow their wheezing as a toddler, it will often occur by about the third or fourth winter. You are not out of the woods yet, though. Some children have wheezing with illnesses as a toddler, outgrow the symptoms for a few years, and then develop allergic asthma when they are 6-8 years old! As you can imagine, this one is quite frustrating for parents.

While the cause of the symptoms is different, the treatment is very much the same. Albuterol for wheezing, controller therapies for persistent/severe symptoms, and systemic steroids for severe symptoms. And don't panic.

Exercise-Induced Asthma and Laryngospasm

Some children can have bronchospasm in response to exercise, even if they have never had asthma symptoms before. If your child experiences exercise-induced asthma, I do not want you taking them out of sports. A large proportion of professional and Olympic-level athletes have asthma. Instead, I want you to find a treatment strategy that will allow your child to continue to enjoy any activity they want. The initial treatment is to use albuterol 15-20 minutes before the activity. This is called "pre-treating," which resolves most patients' symptoms. If the activity lasts longer than 2 hours, repeating the dose is perfectly ok to keep you competing at your best.

A related condition is called Exercise-induced Laryngeal Obstruction

(EILO). This was previously called vocal cord dysfunction, and you may find additional information by searching for this term. EILO is common among athletes. EILO can be confused for exercise-induced asthma, or coexist with exercise-induced asthma. See the comparison below.

In EILO, the vocal cords spasm shut in response to exercise rather than open up to let the air into the lungs. There is no medical treatment for EILO, the proper treatment is to learn breathing techniques that will stimulate your vocal cords to relax and open. There are multiple sources on the internet, and speech therapy can sometimes be helpful to train your child how to relax their airway.

Exercise-Induced Asthma	Exercise-Induced Laryngeal Obstruction
Chest Tightness	Throat tightness
Coughing and wheezing	Stridor and panic
Difficulty on exhalation	Difficulty upon inhalation
Occurs later in exercise, more common long-distance athletes	Occurs soon after onset, more common in sprinters.
More common in long-distance events	More common among sprinters
Lasts 20 minutes untreated	Resolves quickly
Treated with albuterol	Treated with breathing maneuvers

Comorbidities

Your physician will likely ask about other symptoms which can make asthma worse. If your child's nose is congested, it will intensify their symptoms. Even if your child has their asthma completely under control, if there nose is congested they will continue to cough. People who treat asthma will usually also treat nasal congestion since they are so commonly linked. Another common factor is esophageal reflux. Frequent coughing and increased work of breathing can cause esophageal reflux because of the forces occurring inside the body. Since the lungs and food pipe connect at the Adam's apple, stomach acid coming up from the stomach can cause further inflammation in the lungs. Children with asthma and reflux will find that their asthma symptoms improve if the reflux is treated.

Asthma and Anxiety

When people are anxious, they may feel symptoms similar to asthma - namely breathlessness and chest pain. Asthma similarly exacerbates anxiety - it is a terrible feeling to be short of breath. Albuterol can also worsen symptoms of anxiety, since it makes your heart beat faster and can give you jitters.

If anxiety is playing a role in your child's asthma symptoms, consider seeking out a counselor or psychologist in order to treat the anxiety. Controlled breathing exercises may help. One method is to take a slow, deep inhalation through the nose, hold the breath for 2-3 seconds, then exhale fully through pursed lips. Do this multiple times per day and as often as needed.

14

Advocating For Your Child

sthma is a serious condition, and you deserve to have the knowledge and tools in order to care for him/her. There is so much education occurring in a doctor's visit for asthma, that you may not be able to express the questions that are on your mind. You will want to make sure the questions that you do ask are important to you and high yield to help your child.

Here are some topics to consider discussing with your physician:

1. Can you explain my asthma action plan?
2. Who do I call when my child is sick, and when do I go to the emergency room?
3. What side effects should I look for with these medications?
4. Are there any other exposures or conditions that can be making my child's asthma worse?
5. When should I be referred to a specialist (either an allergist or pulmonologist)?
6. I do not believe my child's asthma is under control because of ________.

7. My child has been doing well for months. Is it time to decrease (ie, step-down) the asthma therapies?

Although asthma is common, you will interact with people who do not understand childhood asthma. It is possible your child's babysitter, teacher, or coach will have no experience. Even worse, they may only have had negative experiences with childhood asthma, which will affect how they interact with your child. You should have straightforward conversations with the adults who will be watching your child. Make sure they know he/she has asthma and may need to use their medication or sit and rest at times. Instruct them on signs to look for that your child is having problems. Let them know where the asthma action plan is and how to use it. It would be wise to show them your child's inhaler and how to use it. You are the expert on your child's condition, and you should be prepared to train others how to take care of him/her.

Most children spend the majority of their day at school, and this is a common place for asthma symptoms to occur. Ensure your child's school knows about their condition. Make sure they have an asthma action plan and inhaler (usually with a spacer) for your child. Ask who will give the albuterol when needed - is there a school nurse? Will your child be allowed to carry albuterol on their person? If the school does not have a good plan for your child's safety, ensure they develop one. There is a very good chance your child will miss some school days due to asthma. At the beginning of the school year, ask your child's teacher how make-up assignments and exams will be handled. No child should fail academically because of a poorly timed asthma exacerbation.

15

Conclusion

I sincerely hope this guidebook has helped you understand asthma, its diagnosis, and its treatment. You now know why your child reacts the way he does to colds and other illnesses. You likely have a good idea of what your child's triggers are. Now you will never confuse your controller therapy for albuterol again. Most importantly, you know how to keep your child safe during an attack, on the playing field, and at school.

As I peruse this book, I realize we could discuss many more topics and details. There is always more to know about asthma and health. However, I do not want to overload this quick guide with information that is not useful to you. As a mentor once said:

> *"If your life is a book, asthma should just be a chapter – not the plot."*

If you have found this book helpful, I would greatly appreciate a favorable review at your bookstore of choice so that other parents can find and be helped by this information.

I wish you and your child wellness, success, and love

41

16

References and Resources

FastStats. (2023, Jan 24). Asthma. https://www.cdc.gov/nchs/fastats/asthma.htm

File:Asthma (Lungs).png - Wikimedia Commons. (2016, February 16). https://commons.wikimedia.org/wiki/File:Asthma_%28Lungs%29.png

National Center for Environmental Health. Controlling Asthma in Schools | CDC. (2022, Dec 12). https://www.cdc.gov/asthma/controlling_asthma_factsheet.html

Mheslinga. (2022, Aug 16). Primary care doctors would need more than 24 hours in a day to provide recommended care. University of Chicago News. https://news.uchicago.edu/story/primary-care-doctors-would-need-more-24-hours-day-provide-recommended-care

Mayo Clinic. Prednisone and other corticosteroids. (2022, Dec 9). Mayo Clinic. https://www.mayoclinic.org/steroids/art-20045692

Iannelli, V., MD. (2023). 30 Most Commonly Prescribed Children's Medications. Verywell Health. https://www.verywellhealth.com/the-30-most-prescribed-drugs-in-pediatrics-2633435

Office of the Commissioner. (2020, March 4). Singulair (montelukast) and All Montelukast Generics: Strengthened Boxed Warning - Due to Restricting Use for Allergic Rhinitis. U.S. Food And Drug Administration. https://www.fda.gov/safety/medical-product-safety-information/singulair-montelukast-and-all-montelukast-generics-strengthened-boxed-warning-due-restricting-use

Cleveland Clinic. (2019, Mar 14). Biologic Therapy for Severe Asthma. Cleveland Clinic. https://my.clevelandclinic.org/health/treatments/17711-biologic-therapy-for-severe-asthma

Drugs.com. How to Use A Nebulizer - What You Need to Know. (2023, June 6). Drugs.com. https://www.drugs.com/cg/how-to-use-a-nebulizer.html

CDC - Asthma - Using an Asthma Inhaler Videos. (2022, Dec 12.). https://www.cdc.gov/asthma/inhaler_video/default.htm

Navas, A. (2020, October). When to Go to the ER if Your Child Has Asthma. Nemours Kids Health. Retrieved July 1, 2023, from https://kidshealth.org/en/parents/er-asthma.html

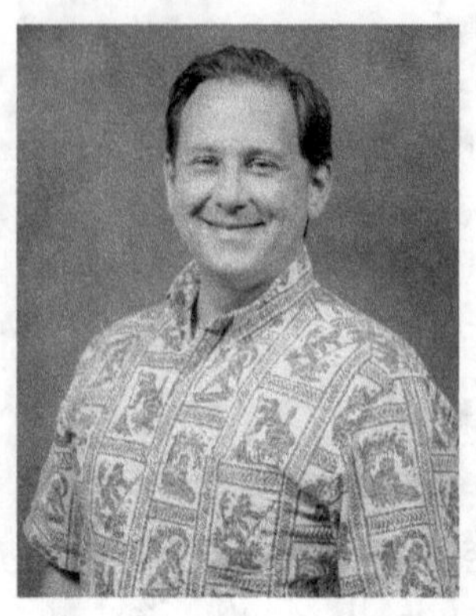

About the Author

Dr. Timothy Beaty is a pediatric pulmonologist working in Honolulu, HI. He has been named to multiple top physician lists, including the Castle Connolly Top Doctors in Honolulu. He has had faculty positions at Emory University, Tulane University, The University of Queensland, and the University of Hawaii. He is also a proud husband and father to four children. When not practicing medicine, Dr. Beaty reads classic literature and plays guitar for the children's ministry at a local church.